ANXIETY ATTACKS

YOU COULD BE A VICTIM

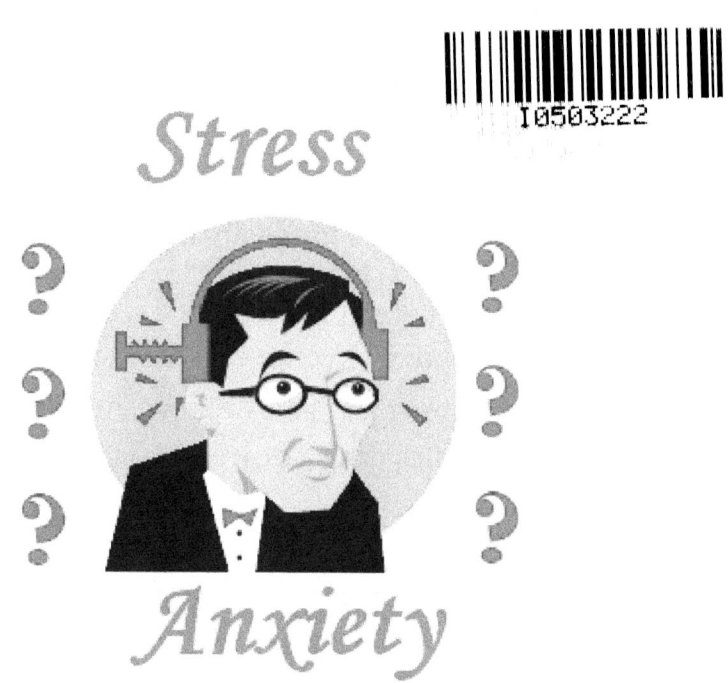

By Patricia A Carlisle

Introduction

I want to thank you and congratulate you for choosing the book, *"ANXIETY ATTACKS: YOU COULD BE A VICTIM"*.

Anxiety attacks, also known as panic attack in emotional or mental wellness circles, are episodes of extreme panic or apprehension. Anxiety attacks are sudden, and can happen at any time and place. This implies that you can frequently feel an attack preceding when it totally hits-sometimes you'll feel a lot of trouble paving the way of the attack before it began.   It can last 10 minutes and it gradually fades through the span of a couple of hours.

Anxiety is the body's common reaction to danger, a programmed alarm that goes off when you feel under pressure, or are confronting a distressing circumstance.

With some restraint, anxiety isn't generally a terrible thing. Anxiety can assist you with staying alert and focused, drive you to action, and rouse you to take care of problems. Yet when anxiety is steady or overpowering, when it disturbs your activities and relationships, and you stop being functional-that is the point at which you've gone too far from ordinary, beneficial or productive anxiety into the area of anxiety disorder or attack.

It's normal to feel restless when confronting a challenging circumstance, for example, an exam, a job interview, or a blind date. But, if your fears and worries appear to be overpowering and interfere with your day by day life, you may be experiencing an anxiety attack. There are various types of anxiety disorders, numerous medications and self-help techniques. Once you understand you have anxiety disorder, there are steps you can take to decrease your symptoms and recapture control of your life.

Thanks again for choosing this book, I hope you enjoy it!

ABOUT THE AUTHOR

Patricia A. Carlisle, MSW, CBT

Patricia Carlisle- a Master Social Worker and Cognitive Behavioral Therapist (CBT) gives out an expression of how important it is for an individual to take into consideration the concept of self-assessment to know what human, technical and conceptual skills they posses to perform or to achieve what they desire, or to deal with everyday life. However, every particular group of people has their own unique set of ideas, traditions and events including the frame of mind according to which people perform but there are many who faces problems and fail to maintain a healthy mind set affecting their behaviors and performance to those around them.

People like Patricia Carlisle are among those who have felt this urge of serving people and helping them out of their mental crisis towards a healthy life. She has experienced some close encounters in her personal life regarding mental health issues in her family and friends that has encouraged her to pursue this as her career.

Currently Patricia Carlisle is serving as a Certified On-Line Cognitive Behavioral Therapist with an extensive 15years of experience using Cognitive-Behavior Therapy Techniques. She envisions a world where everyone gets mental health treatment with no mental health stigma and to make it real she has already set up her own Holistic Measure Online Comprehensive Behavioral Healthcare Company after retiring from The Nord Center in The Partial Hospitalization Program (PHP) Dept for 5 years and Murtis H. Taylor Mental Health Center as a mental health counselor, psychological support technician and case manager for 10 years to emulsify her skills more professionally.

Along with this, she has wrote down her passion as a clinician in 25 or more short books to help individuals and families get their life back, freeing them of the restraints of negative thinking, anxiety and depression by using different approaches. She is highly appreciated among her clients for her flexibility and professionalism of dealing with them graciously. To reach her, make use of her direct website address: http://therapist2013.wix.com/e-therapy . As she is ready to inspire hope and contribute to health and well-being by providing the best online health care through comprehensive practice, education and research.

TABLE OF CONTENT

Chapter 1

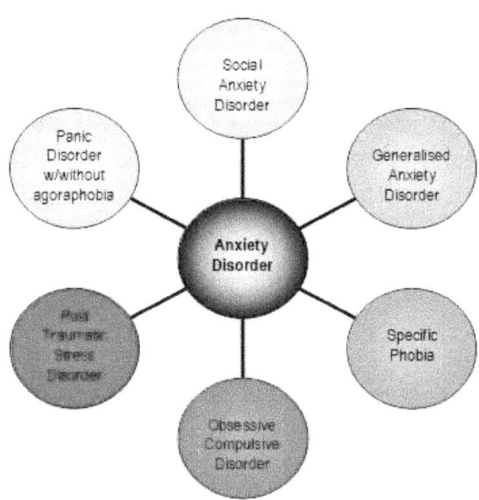

CAUSES OF ANXIETY ATTACKS

An anxiety attack is a physiological reaction of the sympathetic nervous system, which creates the quick acting neurotransmitter adrenaline. Adrenaline makes the signs of an anxiety attack, including fast heart rate, feeling bleary eyed and shortness of breath. Reasons for anxiety attack are situated in mental and biological elements or factors that bring a person to this reaction

PERSONALITY TRAITS

Being a perfectionist or vigilant creates a lot of physical and emotional strain. These generally stable personality characteristics keep the sympathetic nervous system "on lookout." This steady condition of activation expands the risk of an anxiety attack.

COGNITIVE THINKING

Consistent and constant thinking of what could turn out badly or what was left untouched; being excessively worried about future objectives being met keep the sensory nervous system in a condition of arousal, expanding the danger for anxiety attack.

DIATHESIS AND STRESSOR

Biological inclinations that increase the affectability of the sympathetic nervous system, the brain's piece that screens for threats, regularly are known as diathesis. It is a combination of this inclination and particular stressor that makes a person helpless or vulnerable that can increase the danger of a panic attack.

INTENSE STRESS

The sound capacity of the sympathetic nervous system is setting up our body and brain in the time of danger. When we encounter intense stress that overpowers our capacities to cope, (for example, being injured), the reaction from the sympathetic nervous system may trigger a panic attack in a person, rather than sufficiently setting him up to confront the danger.

ANTICIPATORY ANXIETY

Anticipatory anxiety is experienced by the individuals who have panic attacks all the time. This kind of anxiety is a worry of having an anxiety attack. The experience of having an attack is frightening to the point that the individuals who have them add to this continuous worry, which really builds the chances of having another attack.

ADAPTED ANXIETY

Mental conditioning is the process of associating particular events, objects or individuals, with disagreeable emotional states, for example, fear. Once adapted, the mental processes identified with the adapted anxiety, and start to be automatic, and we frequently lack sensitivity of the procedure. For instance, a person who's fear alarm may have developed in childhood, yet not conscious of the occasion that created the condition. They are only mindful of the anxiety, which shows up without any particular reason.

UNDERLYING MEDICAL ISSUES

Medical issues additionally make an affectability, or dysfunction in the sympathetic nervous system. Conditions for example, coronary artery ailment and lupus, are two cases of therapeutic problems that may cause anxiety attack. Additionally, symptoms of some therapeutic conditions can copy signs of an anxiety attack. For instance, vertigo and ear diseases create wooziness or dizziness, which can feel like panic or trigger a panic attack. For those having panic attacks, it is vital to get a medical assessment before you diagnose yourself as having anxiety.

Chapter 2

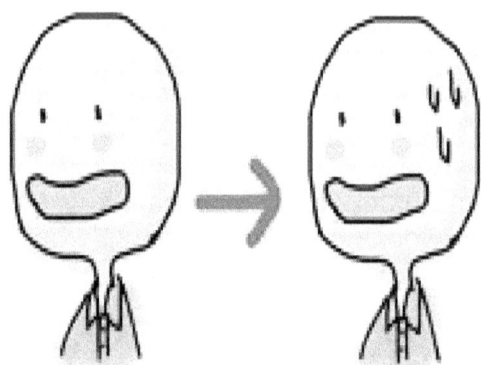

SIGNS AND SYMPTOMS OF ANXIETY DISORDERS

Since anxiety disorders are a gathering of related conditions as opposed to a single disorder, they can look different from individual to individual. One individual may experience the effects of a serious anxiety disorder that strike all of a sudden, while another gets panicky at the thought of joining a group. Another person may battle with the fear of driving, or wild thoughts. Yet another may live in a consistent condition of pressure, agonizing over anything and everything.

In spite of their diverse forms, all anxiety issues constant of serious fear or worry in circumstances where a great many people would feel calm.

EMOTIONAL SYMPTOMS OF ANXIETY

Basic emotional indications of anxiety include:

- Feelings of worry or fear.

- Trouble concentrating.

- Feeling strained and nervous.

- Anticipating the most noticeably bad.

- Irritability

- Restlessness

- Watching for indications of danger.

- Feeling like your mind's not clear.

PHYSICAL SYMPTOMS OF ANXIETY

Anxiety is more than only an inclination or a feeling. As a result of your body's flight and fight reaction, anxiety involves an extensive variety of physical symptoms. In view of the various physical symptoms, anxiety sufferers frequently confuse their disorder for illness. They may visit numerous specialists at health center before there are diagnose with anxiety disorder.

Normal physical symptoms from anxiety include:

- Pounding heart

- Sweating

- Stomach upset

- Frequent urination or loose bowels

- Shortness of breath

- Tremors and jerks

- Muscle tension

- Headaches

- Fatigue

- Insomnia

THE CONNECTION BETWEEN ANXIETY SYMPTOMS AND DEPRESSION

Numerous individuals with anxiety disorder also experience the effects of depression. Anxiety and depression are originated from the same natural vulnerability, which may clarify why they frequently get confused with the other. Since depression exacerbates anxiety (and the other way around), it's vital to look for treatment for both conditions.

Chapter 3

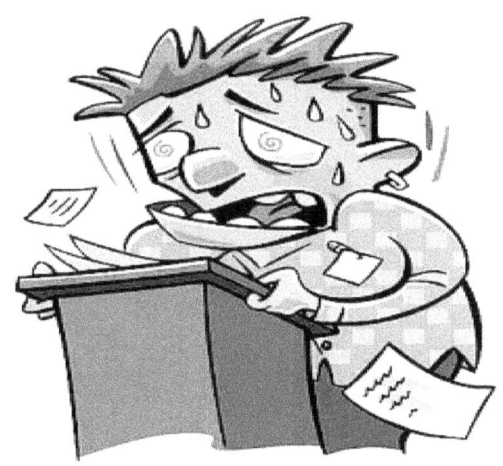

ANXIETY ATTACK AND SYMPTOMS

Anxiety attacks, otherwise called panic attacks, are episodes of extreme fear and panic. Anxiety attacks occur without warning and they are sudden. Some of the time there's a trigger-pondering on an important speech you need to give-yet in different cases, the attacks leave when you are not expected.

Anxiety attacks generally last about 10 minutes, and they sometimes last over 30 minutes. However, in the midst of that brief span, the fear can be severe to the point that you feel as though you're going to die or absolutely lose control. The physical side effects of anxiety attacks are so startling that numerous individuals think they are having a heart attack. After an anxiety attack is over, you may be agonized over thinking you will have another.

SYMPTOMS OF ANXIETY AND ATTACK INCLUDE:

- Surge of overpowering panic.

- Feeling of losing control or going insane

- Heart palpitations or mid-section pain.

- Feeling like you're going to die.

- Trouble breathing or gigging sensation.

- Hyperventilation

- Hot flashes or chills.

- Trembling or shaking.

- Nausea or stomach issues.

- Feeling detached or stunning.

Chapter 4

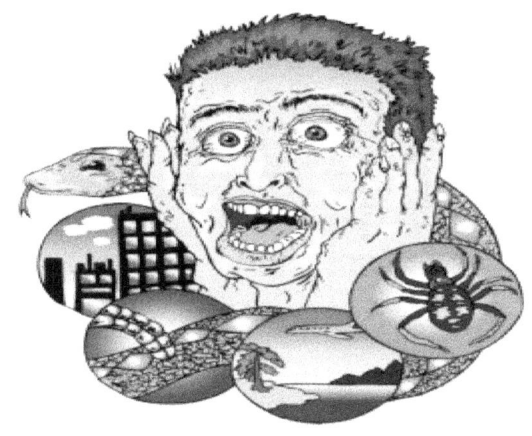

TYPES OF ANXIETY DISORDERS

There are six noteworthy types of disorders, each with their particular unmistakable symptoms:

GENERALIZED DISORDER (GAD)

If steady and consistent fears and worries occupy you from your normal exercises, or you're disturbed by a relentless feeling that something awful is going to happen, you may be experiencing GAD. Individuals with GAD are unending spoilsports who feel restless about everything; meanwhile they may not be shy individuals. Anxiety identified with GAD regularly appears as physical side effects like sleep deprivation, stomach upset, restlessness, and weakness.

PANIC DISORDER

Panic disorder is described by consistent, unforeseen panic attacks, and additionally fears of encountering another episode. A panic disorder might also be joined by agoraphobia, which is the fear of being in places where escape or assist would be a problem in the case of a panic attack. In an event you have agoraphobia, you may want to maintain a strategic distance from public places, for example, shopping centers or restricted spaces, for example, airplane.

OBESSIVE COMPULSIVE DISORDER (OCD)

OCD is described by undesirable thoughts or practices that appear to be difficult to stop or control. If you have OCD, you may be agitated by obsessions, for examples, a repeating worry that you neglected to turn off the stove, or that you may hurt someone. You may also experience the effects of wild compulsions, for example, washing your hands again and again.

PHOBIA

Phobia is an unlikely or misrepresented fear of a particular object, activity, or circumstance that in actuality exhibits next to zero threat. Phobia incorporated fear of creatures (animal); for example, snakes, bugs and also fear of height, and fear of flying. If you are experiencing a serious phobia, you may go to great lengths to maintain a meaningful distance from those things you fear. Tragically, avoidance only reinforces the fear.

SOCIAL ANXIETY DISORDERF (SAD)

If you have a fear of being seen awkwardly by others and humiliated in the public, you may have SAD, and also known as social fear. SAD can be considered as great shyness. In extreme cases, some individuals will stay away from social situations altogether. Stage of performance anxiety (also called fright) is the most widely known type of social fear.

POST TRAUMATIC STRESS DISORDER (PTSD)

PTSD is a compelling anxiety disorder that can happen in the outcome of an unpleasant life event. PTSD can also be referred to as a panic attack that rarely stops. Symptoms of PTSD consist of bad dreams, or flashbacks about what happened, hyper vigilance, startling effectively, pulling back from others, and maintaining a strategic distance from situations that remind you of the event.

Everyone who worries a great deal has an anxiety disorder. You may be anxious because of an excessively requesting timetable, absence of activity or test, pressure at work or at home, or even from drinking too much coffee.

The primary concern is that if your way of life is stressful, you will probably feel anxious-regardless of whether you really have an anxiety disorder. So if you have an inclination that you stress excessively, set aside an opportunity to assess how well you are taking care of yourself.

- Do you set aside a few minutes every day for unwinding and fun?

- Are you getting the emotional support you require?

- Are you dealing with your body?

- Are you over-burdening with obligations?

- Do you request help when you require it?

If your anxiety levels are through the rooftop, consider how you can balance your life. There may be obligations you can give up, turn down, or delegate to others. In case you're feeling secluded or unsupported, find someone you trust. Simply discussing your worries can help you be less anxious.

Chapter 5

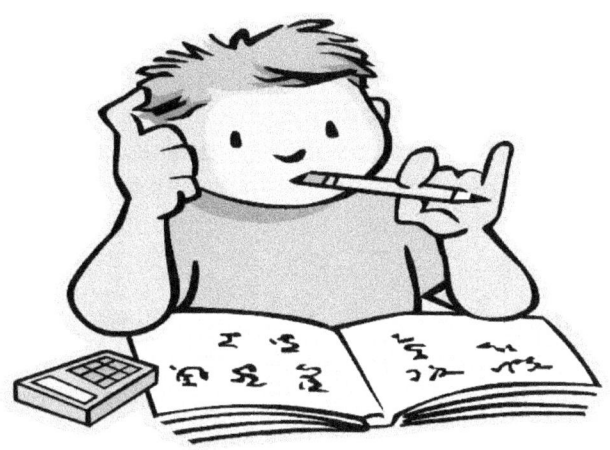

SELF HELP FOR ANXIETY
DISORDERS AND ANXIETY ATTACKS
TEST NEGATIVE THOUGHTS

- **Write down your worries:** Keep paper and pencil on you, or type on a personal computer, cell phone, or tablet. When you encounter anxiety, record your worries. Writing something down is harder work than thinking about them, so you depress your thoughts, and they are prone to vanish sooner.

- **Create an anxiety stress period:** Pick 10-minutes "stress periods" every day that you can commit to anxiety. During your stress period, concentrate just on negative, anxious considerations without attempting to correct them.

- **Accept instability:** Shockingly, agonizing over every one of the things that could turn out badly doesn't make life any more unsurprising-it just keeps you from seeing what you can get out of the great things happening in the present.

TAKE CARE OF YOURSELF

- **Practice unwinding procedures:** Practice frequently unwinding procedures, for example, care contemplation, dynamic muscle unwinding, and breathing can diminish anxiety symptom, and expand feelings of unwinding and emotional prosperity.

- **Adapt to a good diet**: Begin the day with breakfast, and proceed with your regular supper for the duration of the day. Going too long without eating prompts low glucose, and this can make you feel more anxious.

- **Reduce liquor and nicotine:** They prompt more anxiety, not less.

- **Exercise routinely**: Exercise is a characteristic anxiety buster and stress reliever. To accomplish the greatest advantage, go for no less than 30 minutes of high-impact exercise on most days.

- **Get enough rest:** An absence of rest can intensify anxious feelings and thoughts, so attempt to get seven to nine hours of rest a night.

Chapter 6

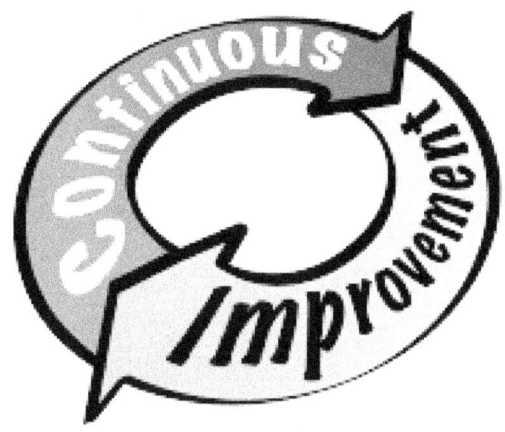

WHEN TO SEEK EXPERT HELP FOR ANXIETY DISORDER

While self-improvement strategies for anxiety can be exceptionally effective, if your fears, worries, or anxiety attack have turned out to be so great that they're bringing about compelling distress, or disturbing your every day schedule, it is imperative to look for expert help.

If you're encountering a great deal of physical anxiety symptoms, think about getting a medical check-up. Your specialist can check to verify that your anxiety isn't brought on by a therapeutic condition, for example, a thyroid issue, hypoglycaemia, or asthma. Since specific medications and supplements can develop anxiety, your specialist will need to take in consideration any medicines, over-the-counter solutions, herbal cures, and recreational medications you're taking.

If your doctor rules out a medical reason, the following step is to talk to an advisor who has experience treating anxiety attacks and anxiety disorders. The specialist will work with you to find the reason, and kind of anxiety disorder and will develop an individual service plan of treatment.

Chapter 7

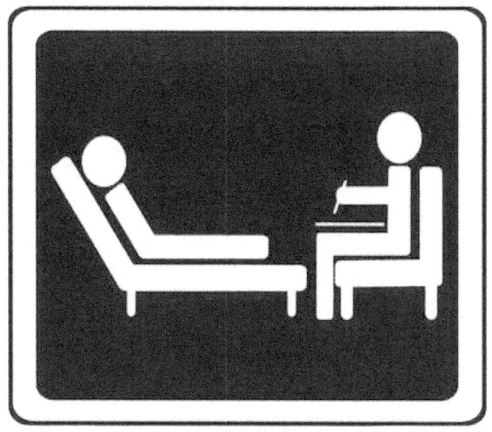

TREATMENT CHOICES FOR ANXIETY DISORDER

Anxiety disorder reacts extremely well to treatment-and frequently in a short measure of time. The treatment approach relies on upon the type of anxiety disorder, and its seriousness. Most anxiety disorder can be treated with behavioral treatment, solution, or some blend of the two. Sometimes alternative and complementary treatments might also be useful.

BEHAVIORUAL TREATMENT FOR ANXIETY DISORDER

Cognitive behavioral treatment and exposure therapy are types of behavioral treatment, which concentrate on conduct as opposed to on basic mental conflicts, or issues from the past. Behavioral treatment for anxiety can take between 5 and 20 week sessions.

- **Cognitive-conduct treatment:** Concentrates on considerations-or cognitions. In anxiety disorder treatment, psychological behavioral treatment assists you with recognizing and testing the negative perception and unreasonable convictions that fuel your anxiety.

- **Exposure treatment:** An anxiety disorder treatment that urges you to go up against your fear in a protected, controlled environment. Through consistent exposures to the dreaded thing or circumstances, either in your creative energy or in reality, you pick up a more prominent feeling of control. As you face your fear without being hurt, your anxiety step by step reduces.

Chapter 8

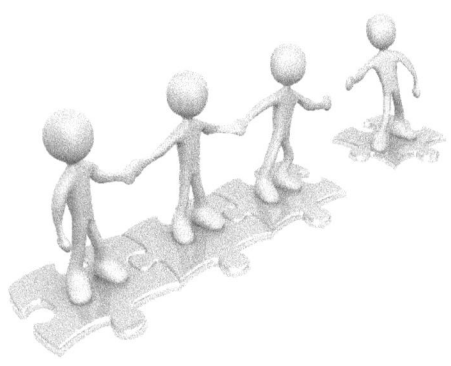

MOST EFFECTIVE METHOD TO HELP SOMEONE EXPERIENCING ANXIETY ATTACK

A person encountering an anxiety attack experiences amazing fear and terror, and may feel as if he or she is having a heart attack. Some individual may experience pain in their mid-section, and hyperventilation. Panic attacks by and large happen all of a sudden, and can reach its peak following 10 minutes, and once in a while last more than 30 minutes.

Here are the following steps to help you or someone else having an anxicty attack:

Step 1: Promise the individual that an anxiety attack is not life debilitating or unsafe. Smoothly clarify that anxiety attack commonly last less than 30 minutes, and promise him or her that you will stay in their vicinity until they feel safe.

Step 2: Try not to ask the individual numerous inquiries, which can bring about extra perplexity. A person encountering an anxiety attack won't have the capacity to process questions properly. Give straightforward answers.

Step 3: Urge the individual to inhale gradually through her nose utilizing medium, not expansive, breaths. Clarify that slow breaths can ease panic attack side effects. If his or her breathing is slow, and they are still complaining about chest pain, they may be experiencing a heart attack, in which case look for prompt emergency therapeutic attention, or call 911. Keep in mind to stay quiet and concentrated regardless of the fact that the circumstance may become severe.

Conclusion

Thank you again for choosing this book!

I hope this book was able to help you to understand and help with your anxiety attacks.

Anxiety attacks are very common in people of all ages. They can range in mild to severity. I hope this information will help you to not become a victim of anxiety disorder and also help those who suffer from anxiety attack to live healthy, happier lives.

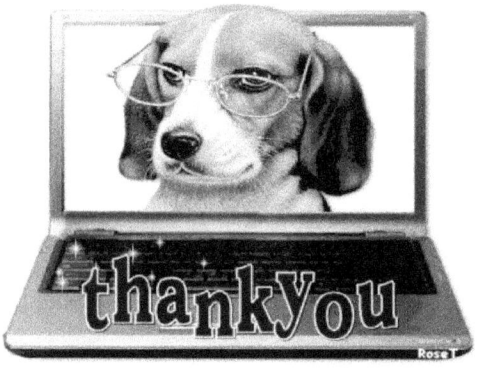

Finally, if you enjoyed this book, would you be kind enough to leave a review for this book on Amazon? It'd be greatly appreciated!

Thank you and good luck!

Preview Of 'Coping with Anxiety Disorder: How to stop Anxiety Tension'

Chapter 1

What is Anxiety Disorder?

Sign, Symptoms and Causes

Among various human emotions, anxiety is one of the most common emotions. It is an emotional or physical turmoil, which can arise from an event or thoughts. Every person in his or her life experiences anxiety or nervousness in many occasions. Our modern life is full of problems, frustrations, time limits and demands. Arguably, stress is not always bad. A person needs anxiety to some extent; it is required for creativity, learning new things and your survival skills. It helps you to be more focused, energetic and prepared. However, when it crosses one's limitation to take stress or it continues for a long period, then it interrupts body's healthy state; it imbalances body's state of equilibrium. Excessive anxiety affects a person's cognitive ability. It can make you feel upset, irritated or worried. In consequence, anxiety starts to cause severe damage to your mind, body, mood, productivity, relationships and quality of your life.

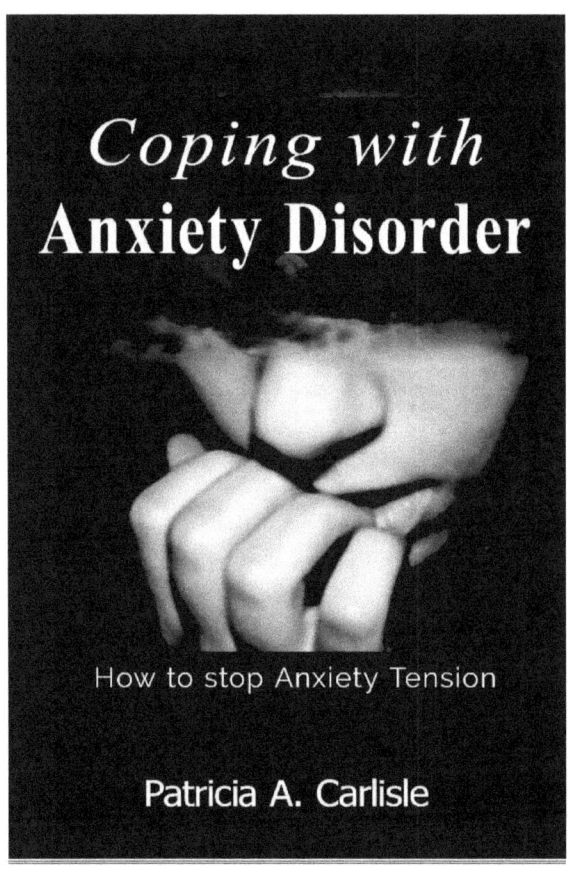

Coping with Anxiety Disorder: How to stop Anxiety Tension.

Check Out My Other Books

Below you'll find some of my other popular books that are popular on Amazon and Kindle as well. Alternatively, you can visit my author page on Amazon to see other work done by me. (https://amazon.com/author/patriciacarlisle)

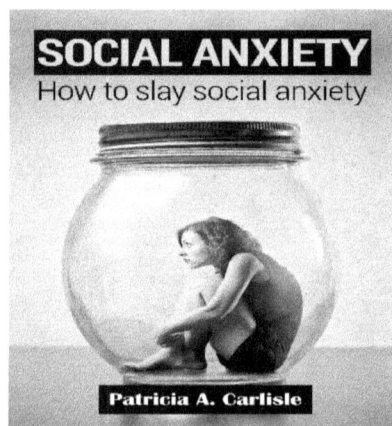

SOCIAL ANXIETY: How to Slay Social Anxiety.

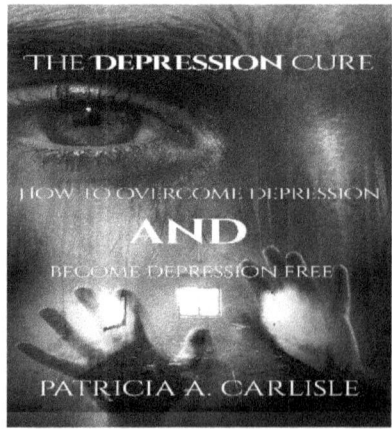

THE DEPRESSION CURE: How to overcome depression and become depression free.

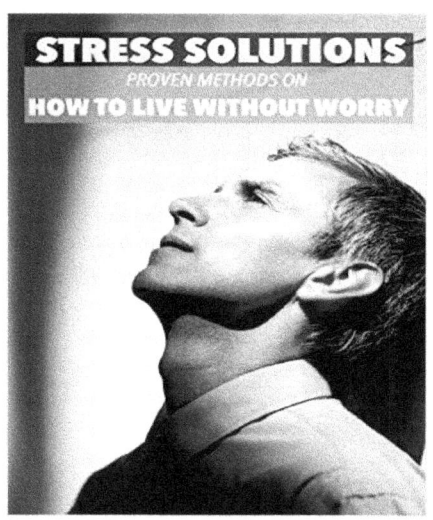

STRESS SOLUTIONS: Proven methods on how to live without worry.

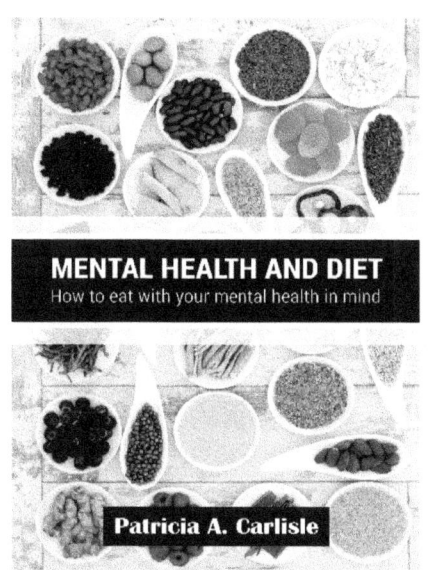

Mental Health and diet: How to eat with your mental health in mind.

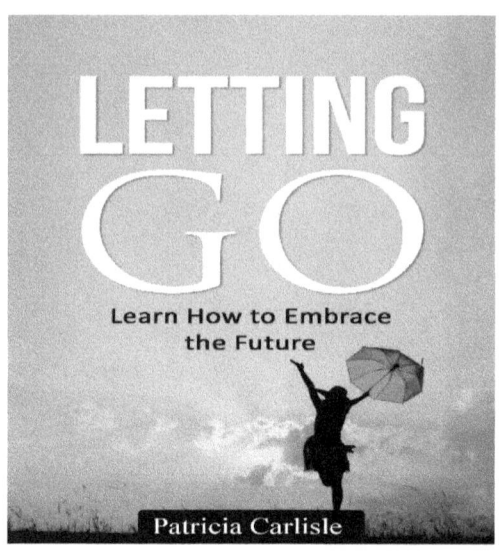

LETTING GO: Learn How to Embrace the Future.

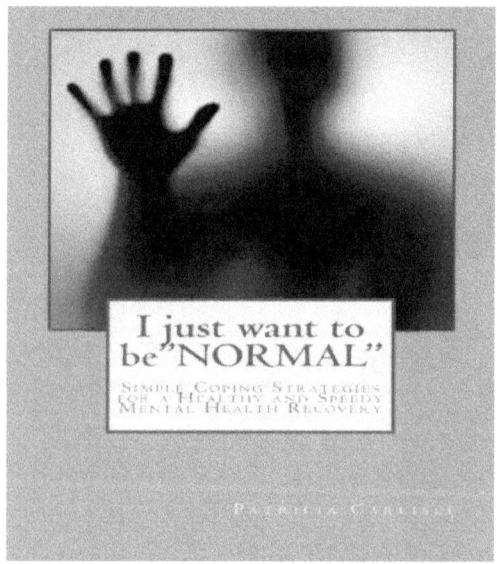

I just want to be "NORMAL" simple coping strategies for a healthier and speedy mental health recovery.

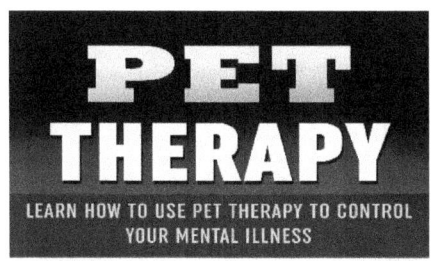
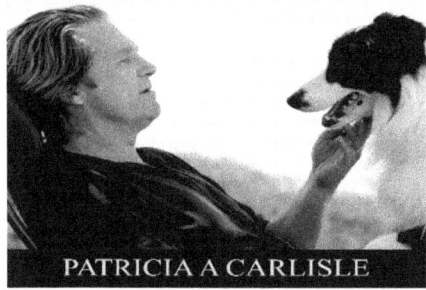

PET THERAPY: LEARN HOW TO USE PET THERAPY TO CONTROL YOUR MENTAL ILLNESS

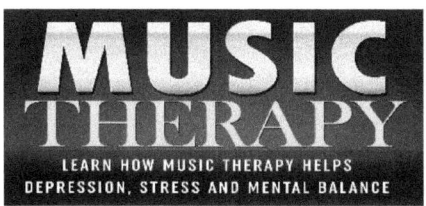
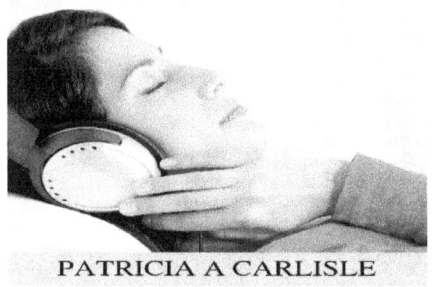

MUSIC THERAPY: LEARN HOW MUSIC THERAPY HELPS DEPRESSION, STRESS AND MENTAL BALANCE.

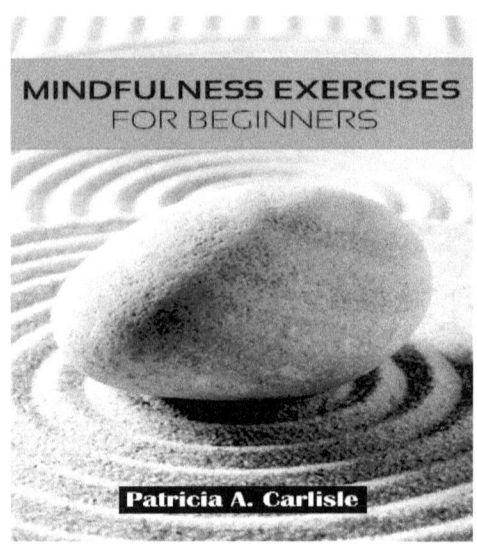

MINDFULNESS EXERCISES FOR BEGINNERS.

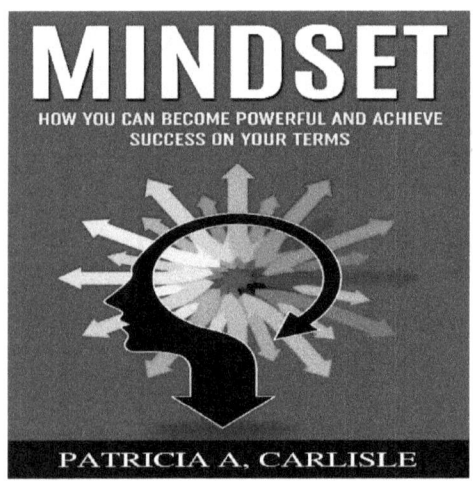

MINDSET: HOW YOU CAN BECOME POWERFUL AND ACHIEVE SUCCESS ON YOUR TERMS.

BONUS: SUBSCRIBE TO THE FREE BOOK

Beginners Guide to Yoga & Meditation

"Stressed out? Do You Feel Like The World Is Crashing Down Around You? Want To Take A Vacation That Will Relax Your Mind, Body And Spirit? Well this Easy To Read Step By Step

E-Book Makes It All Possible!"

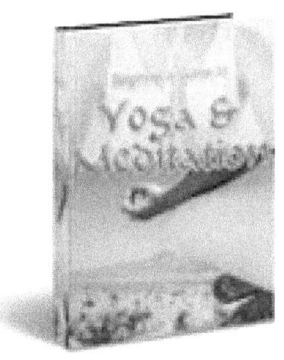

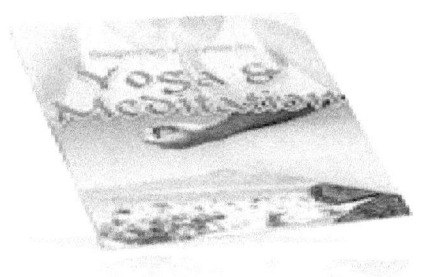

Instructions on how to join our mailing list, and receive a free copy of "Yoga and Meditation" can be found in any of my Kindle eBooks.

NOTES

NOTES

NOTES

NOTES

NOTES

NOTES

NOTES

NOTES

www.ingramcontent.com/pod-product-compliance
Lightning Source LLC
Chambersburg PA
CBHW071012180526
45168CB00003B/1391